Bottom Line on Raspberry Ketones and the Green Coffee Bean Extract Diet A Raspberry Ketone and Green Coffee Bean Extract Supplement Book

Mackenzie Logan

Bottom Line on Raspberry Ketones and the Green Coffee Bean Extract Diet A Raspberry Ketone and Green Coffee Bean Extract Supplement Book

Table of Contents

Brief introduction

Losing weight. Something we all have struggled with one time or another. As difficult as it seems, it need not be. It can be done, and you can achieve the weight you desire. If you are determined to lose your excess weight, I truly believe you will. This book will offer you three ways to reduce the time it takes, and the effort needed to do so. It might just be the answer to your prayers.

The two key methods of weight loss, reducing calorie intake, and increasing calorie usage, (exercise), must be followed. This takes time, and effort. However the good news is there are healthy short-cuts. This book zeroes in on three key supplement short cuts that really work. They really, really work.

I believe that the key to achieving weight loss goals comes through understanding how the supplements work. Once you know and understand, taking them properly is easy. Mistakes won't be made. Success will be achieved, and pounds will fall off and melt away. Forget the hype, forget the false stories of 'I took xyz and one week later lost 28 pounds' and forget the stories saying 'I took xyx and it did nothing for me'. Neither are true. Once you understand the 'why's and how's' of these three supplement short-cuts you'll achieve the results you crave.

We'll start with Raspberry ketone first. (for the sake of easy reading, we'll add an 's' on the end of Raspberry ketone to make it easy to understand, but correctly speaking, it should not be pluralized like that).

Raspberry Keytones

Taking Raspberry ketones supplements is an excellent way of losing weight. Raspberries have always been considered to be one of the healthiest fruits available. Keytones are primary compounds that are found in raspberries and are known for burning fat in the body without any side effects. They also have other health benefits such as enhancing immunity and improving the skin.

If you have ever tried to lose weight previously, then you probably know by now how difficult the process is and how exhausting it can be to find an effective diet supplement. A new supplement is being released every day and the truth is that most of them don't work. The worst thing that can happen is you waste your time and money on a product that doesn't work, especially if you have been trying really hard to lose weight for a long time. What makes it even more stressful is that there are various scams going on right now, whether it is online or in retail stores. There are thousands of products in the market right now that promise fast and effective results, but unfortunately this is not what happens in the end.

Fad diets, diet plans, vigorous exercises, and dieting are all going to find a way into the lives of individuals who are trying to lose weight at some point. However, this doesn't mean that their efforts will pay off or that the diet or pills will work. Many diets and pills fail most of the time, and this will leave you with excess weight and a spirit that it broken. Breaking away from this cycle is very important if you are trying to live a life that is healthy. This is one of the best things about the diets mentioned in this book. Users won't have to worry about any side effects and they will help you in reaching the ideal weight and body shape you were wishing for.

Most of the diets mentioned in this book have been gaining a lot of popularity during the previous months, ever since Dr. Oz introduced some of these diets on his show. Dr. Oz is one of the trusted professionals in the field and he has the described them as the 'world's miracle for losing weight'. The Raspberry ketone diet, for example, is a supplement used for weight loss that only consists of raspberry ketones and other natural components. Not only is the diet used for weight loss, but it was also proven to have other health benefits, such as increasing metabolism and decreasing the risk of cancer. These diets are considered to be one of the top sellers amongst weight loss supplements and are used by thousands of people from different areas of the world. The purpose of this book is to explain the components of these diets, how they work, and the various benefits of using them. You will also be able to understand the best blends and sources to purchase them from, along with how you can increase the effects of the diet in a fast and effective manner.

About a Supplement called Raspberry Ketones

Raspberry ketones are aromatic and organic components that are found in raspberries and various other fruits. Ketones are responsible for the outstanding smell of raspberries. This is why they used in several perfumes and during cooking as well. Research has proven that ketones lead to weight loss as they consist of compounds that increase the body temperature and in turn enhance metabolism. This will increase the body's metabolism rate and this is why fats are burnt at a faster rate.

Raspberries have always been considered to be one of the healthiest fruits available. Supplements and diets that consist of raspberry ketones harness unique properties that promote weight loss. When this diet is follow properly, it can help individuals in losing weight easily and solving other weight management problems. This is due to raspberry ketones playing an important role in enhancing metabolism, one of the most important benefits of following this diet as well. When the process of fat absorption is reduced in the body, this will also result in the reduction in the amount of fat and other toxins stored in the body.

Even though they are completely natural, they are also produced in different labs around the world synthetically. What a lot of people aren't aware of is that raspberry ketones are also available in various other fruits such as cranberries or blackberries. The original compound is biosynthesized from the chemical coumaroyl-CoA. The process of extracting raspberry ketone is done using one to four mg per kg of different types of raspberries. Since raspberry ketones aren't naturally abundant all the time, many companies prepare ketones industrially using various chemical intermediates. On the plus side, these biosynthesized versions work just as well as eating the pounds and pounds of raspberries you would need to consume to gain the same weight loss goal. Even raspberry ketone products that claim to be '100%' natural are made this way.

Scientists have already proven that the pungent compounds in raspberry ketones are capsaicin, lipolytics, and synephrine. They are the main reason behind the breakdown of fats. In an experiment that was conducted, rats were fed food that was high in fat for ten weeks. Researchers made the observation that when the rats were injected with raspberry ketone, the amount of fat around their liver and tissues was automatically decreased. Scientists also observed that the amount of fat surrounding vitro cells decreased and a higher amount of adiponectin was secreted. Raspberry ketones also consist of components that reduce the amount of excess fat that is normally absorbed in the body. During the past few years, nutritionists and fitness trainers would suggest consuming a diet that contains raspberries and this just proves how effective this diet is.

Components of Top Grade Raspberry Ketones Supplement and their Benefits

Before you start using this outstanding supplement, it is essential that you understand its components first. To lose weight effectively, there are other great components in the supplement that you should be aware of such as:

•African mango is another important component in this diet and its benefits include controlling cravings, which helps the body to burn excess fat at a faster rate. African mango also assists in increasing the rate of metabolism in the body, which results in excess fat transforming to energy quicker. When the metabolism in your body is stabilized, this will result in you having more energy. This is very beneficial for individuals who have anaemia or suffer from having low energy levels.

•Acai berry consists of antioxidants that the body needs to function properly. During the process of weight loss, our body needs various vitamins, minerals, nutrients, and anti-oxidants to stay healthy. Consuming acai berries also results in the body balancing the homeostasis levels in the body. This includes balancing hormones that are responsible for stabilizing the fat levels in your body, so this is definitely beneficial if you are trying to love weight. Acai berries also contain antioxidants that reduce any excess fat absorption in the body.

•Resveratrol consists of antioxidants that can be used to protect the heart from any risks of coronary diseases. Resveratrol has been used for years in the prevention of serious diseases such as Alzheimer, diabetes and cancer.

•Apple cider vinegar has been used for years to help individuals in losing weight effectively. Apple cider vinegar is beneficial in restoring acid levels in the digestive system that are responsible for breaking down any excess fats or proteins. This makes the body able to digest the food you eat more easily. This results in your body absorbing nutrients more easily and in turn this results in your body being stronger and healthier. Another great benefit of cider vinegar is that you will be able to control any food cravings you have. Recent research has shown that regular consumption of cider vinegar will decrease levels of triglyceride and body fat.

•Green tea is extracted from a plant known as carellia sinesis. Green tea is also known for having strong medicinal powers that can protect you from high blood pressure, unstable cholesterol levels, and headaches. It was found that individuals who use green tea on a regular basis have a very low risk of developing diseases such as diabetes or high cholesterol. Green tea is also very beneficial for your teeth as it consists of antibacterial chemicals and fluoride, substances that are essential in preventing any type of gum diseases or cavities. It was also found that consuming regular quantities of green tea on a regular basis will decrease your risk of suffering from Alzheimer's and Parkinson's disease.

•Caffeine is another important component of this diet. The first advantage of caffeine is that it can decrease your risk of suffering from cancer or Parkinson's disease. Caffeine also decreases your risk of suffering from diabetes, especially among women. A previous research was conducted for cancer patients, where powder was applied on their skin and they were later exposed to UV rays. After the test was finished, most cancer tumors were reduced by 70%. Most medical professionals believe that this is due to caffeine blocking ATR proteins, the main reason behind the increase in the size of tumors.

•Grapefruit is one of the essential providers of nutrients and vitamin C. Vitamin C is very important for strengthening the immune system and relieving any sicknesses. It can also be used to relieve breathing problems, especially when it comes to asthma. Grapefruit is full of enzymes that assist the body in breaking down fats and this is why many people consume it to lose weight. The smell of grapefruit decreases cravings and this prevents any type of overindulging or excess eating. Grapefruit also consists of salicylic acid that breaks down inorganic calcium in the body and builds healthy join cartilage. Individuals who consume grapefruit on a regular basis are less prone to diseases such as arthritis. Grapefruit is an excellent germ killer as well and is used to treat fungal contaminations like candida and herpes.

•Kelp is a sea vegetable that many people aren't aware of. It is abundant in many nutrients and is high in iron. It aids the body in the digestion process and purifies from any unhealthy radiation. Even though it is usually used by women during pregnancy, it is also an excellent supplement for weight loss.

Raspberry Ketone enzymes are the main ingredients in this diet and they are the main reason behind the weight loss that many people experience. The health benefits of raspberry ketones will be covered in the next chapter.

The best raspberry ketones supplements will consists of the following components:

•Raspberry Ketone extract (4%) 300 mg

•Green Tea (50% extract) 200 mg

•Caffeine Anhydrous 100 mg

•Proprietary blend 600 mg Consisting of: Apple Cider Vinegar (powder), Grapefruit (powder), Kelp, Acai Fruit (powder), African Mango (4:1 concentrate), Resveratrol Extract.

Even though the dosages may differ from one company to another, you should ensure that the raspberry ketone diet you consume consists of these ingredients so you can be able to lose weight effectively.

How does the Supplement Work On Your Body To Result In Weight Loss?

Raspberry ketone is a natural and healthy component that is found in all type of raspberries. This makes them 100% safe to use and this is one of the few diets that can be used without worrying about any side effects or risks. Contrary to what many people believe, we are born with the same amount of cells that consist of fats and we will die with the same amount as well. When people gain weight, this will result in the fat and other cells increasing in their size. Oppositely, when we lose weight, this will result in the same cells decreasing in their size.

When you think about it, this is the main reason why most invasive surgeries such as liposuction don't work permanently. When these fat cells are removed, our body will innately respond to this change by the increasing the amount of fat cells that we originally had. Instead of spending thousands of dollars on surgeries that only have only temporary results and have a high possibility of failure, it is recommended to use a natural raspberry ketone supplement and exercise. Not only will this accelerate the weight loss process, but you also won't have to worry about any risks that are threatening to your life.

Raspberry ketones work by breaking down the fat cells in our body in an effective manner. This will help you in burning any excess fat at a faster rate. Raspberry ketones also influence the adiponectin hormones in the body. These hormones trick the body into thinking it is thin when they are excreted. Research has proven that individuals who aren't overweight and have a normal body shape have a very high amount of the hormone adiponcetin, and this is why it is usually easier for them to burn fat quicker.

On the other hand, individuals who are overweight have extremely low amount of the adiponectin and this is why it is easier for their body to store excess weight. Adiponectin hormones also shrink the fat cells in your body by increasing its ability to burn fats. It has various anti-inflammatory features that protect the heart and have a very strong influence on the body's response in excreting insulin.

Additionally, raspberry ketones are known to increase your metabolism. Research has proven that this supplement is able to stabilize metabolism in a way that wasn't displayed by other supplements previously. This takes place by increasing your body's temperature and this is why individuals who use this diet are able to lose weight quickly. Metabolism is also increased by breaking down the lipids in your body into smaller components known as fatty acids. These fatty acids are then used for the production of energy in your body.

If you follow this supplement usage properly, you will be able to lose up to three to six pounds per week. This will differ between one person to another depending on various factors such as their body shape, whether they are suffering from health problems or not, and if they are using other techniques along with the diet, such as exercising. The recommended dosage would be twice per day; once during breakfast and another dosage after lunch. If you decide to use the 50mg dosage pills, then you might have to increase your dosage to four times per day. Don't take this supplement too late, or it make keep you awake. Lack of sleep inhibits weight loss and hurts the immune system.

If you conduct research online, you will find thousands of positive reviews from previous customers who have followed the supplement and were able to lose weight successfully. If you don't trust customer reviews, you should check clinical trials and testimonials from the best doctors in the world so you can get convinced how great this product really is.

It has already been verified countless times that Raspberry ketone supplements actually work and will speed up your weight loss. It is essential that you understand that results will be different from one person to another and this is due to several factors such as body shape and overall health. For example, you will find someone losing four pounds per week and another person might be able to lose more than that. This will also depend on the diet you are following and whether you are exercising while you are consuming the diet.

Benefits of using the Raspberry Ketones Supplement

As stated previously, the raspberry ketone diet was tested several times through extensive clinical trials. Raspberry ketones are rated as GRAS by the FDA which means that they are 'generally recognized as a safe product.' A study that was conducted by the clinic Morimoto et al examined the effects of Raspberry ketones on rats that were overweight. The rats that were fed raspberry ketones and fatty food lost weight whereas the ones who were fed fatty food only didn't lose any weight at all. Results have also shown that enzymes in raspberries substantially decrease any possibility of weight gain from consuming a diet that is high in fats, however that is not recommended. Additionally, the enzymes also decrease any fat accumulation that can take place around the kidneys and liver.

There are several other benefits that users should be aware of such as:

Benefit #1: Research has confirmed that consuming raspberries on a regular basis can assist the body in excreting a specific protein that is responsible for burning fats. This is a special protein that is also responsible for enhancing the efficiency of the immunity system and other metabolic processes. When the body excretes this protein, this will significantly eliminate any fat components in your body, resulting in you losing excess weight. Additionally, this protein is also responsible for regulating glucose levels. Without doubt, one of the main reasons why people use this diet is to lose weight. This diet is becoming the best way to lose weight and burn fats in a healthy and safe manner. When it is combined with other products such as African mango, users will be able to lose weight in a faster manner and improve their skin condition and immune system as well.

Benefit #2: Consuming this diet can regulate cholesterol levels and stabilize blood pressure. This is very beneficial for individuals who are older in age and are suffering from health problems. This is an important benefit for your body because other diets achieve the same effect but the only difference is that your cardiovascular system will be affected negatively. This is not the case with the raspberry ketones diet.

Benefit #3: The diet has purportedly worked in curing and preventing various types of cancer. Research has proven that enzymes in raspberries consist of anti-carcinogenic features that will protect your esophagus, liver, skin, and colon from cancer. The enzymes are also very rich in different phytochemicals such as elegiac acid which reduces your risk of suffering from cancer.

Benefit #4: The raspberry ketone diet consists of natural antioxidants and chemicals that can greatly protect your skin and cells. There is no doubt that antioxidants are very important especially that we are always prone to damaging effects from free radicals. Right now, there are free radicals that are harmful everywhere around us and this diet can protect your cells from any damages. This is very important because free radicals are known to greatly speed up the aging process and might be the trigger of various serious illnesses. The diet also gives your skin a healthy glow that is rarely achieved with other types of diets.

Benefit #5: The diet has also proven to alleviate inflammation and decreases the pain associated with arthritis or gout. The anti-inflammatory features of the diet are somewhat similar to aspirin and various other anti-inflammatory medications. There is no doubt that arthritis and gout can be extremely painful and stressful. Consuming this diet will also be extremely beneficial for individuals who exercise while following this diet and want to prevent muscular pain as much as possible. It will also ensure that individuals who suffer from gout don't have the same amount of digestion or swallowing problems.

Benefit #6: Raspberries are known in assisting the metabolic systems in releasing omega-3 acids. Omega-3 acids are essential for preventing any skin ailments. They also play an important role in enhancing brain functions and releasing growth hormones. This is the main reason why most fitness and dieting experts advise their clients to consume foods that have a high percentage of omega-3 acids.

Benefit #7: The raspberry ketone diet consists of supplements that are 100% natural. This means that users don't have to worry about suffering from side effects, unlike other diets or pills that are known for having negative effective on the body. There aren't any artificial ingredients added to the product which makes it extremely safe and effective in improving your overall health as well. Keep in mind that most diet pills are known for having serious side effects on the health, such as kidney or liver damage.

Benefit #8: The raspberry ketone diet plays an important role in reducing the amount of cellulite in the body. Cellulite is a problem that faces many people especially women and results in them facing challenges with their self-confidence and esteem. This is very important especially for women who usually look for a diet that will improve their overall body shape as well.

Benefit #9: One of the most important benefits of the raspberry ketone diet is that food cravings will be controlled. The main reason why many people can't lose weight is because they can't control the amount of food they consume per day or feel that they have any control over eating. However, this soon stops because food cravings will be controlled. People find that they don't feel hungry all the time.

Benefit #10: Due to the fact that raspberries consist of natural minerals, it can decrease the feeling of nausea. Many people experience irritation in their stomach lining when they are trying to lose weight but this won't happen to them when they consume this diet. This is also important for individuals who suffer from digestion problems or constipation.

Benefit #11: Cost is one of the factors that many people look at before they purchase a weight loss supplement or diet, especially if they are on a tight budget. Even though raspberry ketone diets are a bit more expensive that other products, if you compare it to other weight loss techniques such as liposuction, you will find that it is very affordable and you will probably be able to purchase a year worth of products instead of paying for a surgery at 50 times the cost and which has temporary and irreversible side effects.

Introduction of the Pure Green Coffee Bean Extract Diet

Another great supplement you can use to lose weight is green coffee beans extract. The main source of green coffee beans are plants known as Arabica. Arabica plants consist of a higher chlorogenic acid percentage, which is why many people prefer using them instead of other plants. However, it can also be extracted from raw beans and seeds. During their production, the beans will usually have to be extensively brewed first before they can be used. Many manufacturers avoid roasting them because this will destroy the important compounds inside them. Even though many people have tried using different types of ordinary coffee for losing weight, this method does not work properly and some people even ended up suffering from side effects and withdrawal symptoms. It has been proven several times that green coffee extract is much better and doesn't have any side effects.

The pure green coffee bean diet is another outstanding supplement that was promoted by Dr. Oz in his television show. This supplement represents all the latest nutritional research and the best thing about it is that it is also available in the form of capsules. The product was endorsed various times publicly by some of the best medical professionals in United States and other areas of the world. This is a product that has helped people not only lose weight, but improve their health in different ways. This is very important because users of this outstanding weight loss supplement will result in reaping two benefits at the same exact time.

Pure green coffee is completely different from brown coffee and this was a point that confused many people in the beginning. Brown coffee is usually roasted at 470 degrees, whereas green coffee beans aren't because this will completely destroy the enzymes inside them. This is also why they have a completely different flavor and aroma. They usually have a bitter taste and medical professionals have stated many times that the more bitter the green coffee beans are, the better they are. They also consist of 50% cholorogenic acid, and this is the main substance behind the weight loss that many people experience.

For several years now, there was a very strong debate on whether green coffee extract can be used effectively for weight loss or not. Research that will be explained in the next chapters has proven that green coffee beans consist of properties that are extremely beneficial for weight loss and your overall health. The beans can also enhance metabolism in a way that isn't found in most other metabolism boosters. It is an outstanding source of energy that will have outstanding effects on your attempt to lose weight.

Medical professionals and researchers were very impressed with the fact that the extract of coffee beans is very nutritional as well. This means that they don't have to be mixed with any other drugs or fillers before they are sold to customers. This is why it is now used by thousands of people all over the world right now, as well as countless others who stopped after achieving their weight loss goals.

How does the Supplement Work and Lead to Weight Loss?

Green coffee beans consist of the natural compound chlorogenic acid and fiber. These are the main components of green coffee bean extract that lead to weight loss. There are three different types of fiber in coffee beans and cellulose. Chlorogenic acid burns fats in the body by inhibiting glucose utilization. This is very important as excess glucose along with fats is the main reason behind gaining weight. When there isn't any excess sugar in the body, this means that fats won't build up in the body and you will be able to lose weight more effectively.

Green coffee beans also consist of antioxidants that have other health benefits such as eliminating free radicals and other toxins from the body. Chlorogenic acid boosts the metabolism in our body and this prevents any excess fat from becoming stored in the body, especially around the liver. This is why many people experience a boost in their energy when they start taking green coffee bean extract supplement. This is very important because our liver is responsible for processing fats in the body. Keep in mind that high sugar levels in the body can result in weight gain and the increase of toxins and radicals in our body. Cholorgenic acid in green coffee bean extracts will be able to break down any other toxins in your body in an effective manner as well. This will also help ensure that your body can fight off serious diseases.

Studies and research conducted

One of the most important studies that was done on coffee bean extract was the one by Dr. Joe Vinson and Bryan Burnham. This study involves a focus group of sixteen individuals who were overweight. They were given coffee bean extract on a daily basis along with a diet of 2000 calories. Although the amount of calories is higher than the amount that is recommended, none of them exercised and they were still able to lose weight. Over twelve weeks, they were able to lose approximately seventeen pounds. This weight loss was 10.5% of their overall weight and 16% of their body fat. This was a finding that impressed researchers at the time as they didn't expect them to lose weight at all during such a short time.

A further study was conducted by Japanese researchers during 2005. The study involved various participants who were given green coffee bean extract. Some of these participants suffered from hypertension. This study was completely different from the others as its purpose was to examine the health benefits of green coffee bean extract and not whether it results in weight loss or not. The results were very impressive. The participants didn't experience any side effects and their hypertension problems decreased. Many participants also experienced stabilization in their cholesterol levels.

Another important research that was conducted was by Dr. Oz himself. The medical unit of his show select 100 random women who were between 35 to 50 years old. Almost all of these women were also overweight and their body mass indexes were 35 to 55. None of these women were pregnant, breastfeeding, or suffering from serious medical issues, such as diabetes and heart attacks. All the women received any equal 400mg dosage of green coffee bean extract capsules. They were informed to take them three times per day, half an hour before every meal. They were informed to be avoiding missing a dosage as this will slow down the process of losing weight and will lead to the results of the research being incorrect.

None of these women changed their diet and kept on eating the same way they naturally did. They also kept a food journal so the medical unit working for the Dr. Oz show would have an idea about the food they were consuming. After three weeks, the participants returned and were weighed. It was found that most of these women lost two to three pounds. The women who lost even more than average, was due to consuming food that was lower in fat. This is why Dr. Oz advised his viewers to be careful of what they eat and try to exercises as much as they can as well. Overall, he proved that this weight loss supplement is very effective in weight loss. Dr. Oz was very impressed with the results and this is why he immediately started recommending it to all his viewers.

Other studies that were conducted whether on animals or humans have similar results as well. Unanimously, professional researchers have concluded that green coffee extract is one of the most effective and safe ways to lose weight. Thousands of medical professionals from all over the world have recommended individuals who are trying to lose weight to use it. It is sold by a lot of companies and is usually in the form of capsule which makes it very easy to take.

Recommended Dosage

It is recommended that the daily dosage of the green coffee bean diet is 800 mg per day. To reach the desired effects, the dosage should be taken two times per day, once before breakfast and another time after dinner. You should try to stick to a schedule to avoid any confusion. Professionals advise to avoid taking the supplement with food and they should take it thirty minutes prior to eating with a glass of water. This will also help the body in staying hydrated and burning excess fats. You will find many different companies that offer green coffee bean extract supplements, but you need to understand several aspects regarding the ingredients first before you choose. You should never be duped by products that are ineffective and you should always play close attention to the ingredients in the supplement. When you find a company that you trust, you should ensure that the supplement consists of the following ingredients:

•GCA®. These are the antioxidants in the extract that lead to all the health benefits.

•Svetol®. This is the ingredient that has very strong inhibitory actions on the absorption of glucose in your diet. It also modulates all the factors that are needed for absorbing sugar from diets.

•Cholorgenic acid. It is essential that the capsule consists of at least 45% chlorogenic acid. Even though a higher percentage will be okay, you should ensure that the percentage isn't less to ensure that you will reap all the health benefits and lose weight effectively.

You should note that the capsules will differ depending on their dosage. You will find capsules that have 200mg, 400mg, and even 800mg. Even though these dosages differ, they will all result in you losing weight but you should make sure that you take a dosage that is suitable for your health and body condition. It is advisable to purchase a food journal, so you can monitor the amount and types of food you consume. Even though you will end up losing weight when you use green coffee bean extract, this doesn't mean that you should eat anything you want. You should try as much as possible to eat foods that are low in fat and eat plenty of vegetables along with drinking water. Be smart!

Benefits of the Green Coffee Bean Extract Diet

Benefit #1: Green coffee beans are effective in eliminating free radicals. Free radicals usually increase in the body due to various reasons, such as poor digestion or disease. They can lead to serious problems and can damage our immune system, increase our risk of suffering from cancer, and speed up the aging process. The chlorogenic acid in green coffee bean extract consists of antioxidants that fight free radicals through absorbing them. This will decrease the amount of fat cells generated in your body. Eliminating free radicals is very important to ensure that your overall health condition is in great shape as well.

Benefit #2: Coffee bean extract consists of chlorogenic acid, which inhibits enzymes such as glucose-6-phosphate that are responsible for releasing glucose into our bloodstream, especially when we consume meals. The extract will assist the body in regulating levels of glucose and will decrease your risk of suffering from diabetes. Keep in mind that stable glucose levels have a lot of benefits such as slowing the aging process, decreasing inflammation, and detoxification of the body. This is one of the few products that anyone can take no matter if they suffer from diabetes or not.

Benefit #3: Chlorogenic acid increases metabolism in your body and this will enable the liver to break down fats easier and will help you in losing weight effectively. Fats will also be absorbed at a slower rate and this will aid weight loss as well. Chlorogenic acid also encourages a process known as thermogenesis that involves the body burning fat in exchange of energy. When thermogenesis takes place effectively, excess fat in your body will be burnt quickly. This will definitely enable you to lose weight at a faster rate.

Benefit #4: Green coffee bean extract can also decrease hypertension. Research that was conducted by the Japanese corporation Kao revealed very positive effects on humans and animals that suffered from mild hypertension. The research demonstrated decreased levels of blood pressure in both humans and animals. The greater the dosage they took, the better the results were.

Benefit #5: Consuming green coffee bean extract has no side effects and this is very important as most weight loss techniques have serious side effects on your health and body. Many other weight loss products and diet pills have resulted in their users suffering from serious health problems, such as shaking, nausea, and mood changes. Chlorogenic acid on the other hand results in individuals losing weight by interrupting the release of excess glucose, which is completely safe.

Benefit #6: Improves your cardiovascular health as chlorogenic acid has proven to decrease cholesterol and blood pressure levels. There is no doubt that your cardiovascular health is very important and taking this supplement will improve it. You will also notice that your breathing problems will have diminished if you are suffering from any.

Benefit #7: Due to green coffee bean extract consisting of ingredients that boost metabolism, you energy levels will increase. This is extremely beneficial for individuals who have anaemia or deficiency in other nutrients. Recently, Starbucks has launched new products that consist of a range of green coffee. They promote the increasingly well-known medical benefits of green coffee. This is the perfect supplement to take especially after a very tiring day of working or studying.

Benefit #8: Green coffee extracts are effective colon cleansers and can stabilize bowel movements. This is beneficial for individuals who suffer from constipation or other similar problems. This will also decrease your risk of suffering from problems such as colon or liver cancer. When your colon is clean, this has other health benefits as well such as increasing healthy bacteria in your intestine and enhancing the immunity system.

Benefit #9: This is one of the few supplements that can be used by all adults no matter what their health condition or age is. Even though research has proven that it has no side effects on children, it is advised that only people who are above 18 should take it.

Bonus Section: Brazilian Acai berry Diet Supplements

Nature does her magic again! In ancient times man used to depend on nature for his food, medicine, clothes and all basic needs. Today, it is no different! People tend to use the fruits and herbs provided by Mother Nature, as food and even for medicinal purposes. The Brazilian Acai berry is just another example of such a blessing from Mother Nature, which has been gaining huge popularity for its use in weight loss supplements. Like the different weight loss supplements available in the market today, the Brazilian Acai berry is another great supplement that you can use to lose weight. Let us go to the history of these berries and understand how they proved so beneficial for weight loss.

The fruit originates from a palm tree species, mainly found in floodplains and swamps. A blackish purple round fruit, the Acai berry resembles a grape fruit, but smaller than it, with lesser flesh. Used by the tribal people in the jungles of Amazon, these berries soon became popular for their healing properties for different diseases. It was these tribal people who discovered the qualities of the Acai berry and found that it had the ability to reduce bad cholesterol, strengthen the immune system and provide a lot more benefits, which would be of immense help to mankind.

This extract from the rainforests of Brazil is today well-known for having antioxidants and improving the immune system of humans. Not only does it reduce the amount of bad cholesterol in our body, but its consumption also aids in the increase of the good cholesterol level too, thereby keeping our body in a perfectly healthy condition that is devoid of all excess fats.

For those people who spend hours and hours in a gym or for those who tire themselves out walking long stretches every day, this berry comes as a blessing and a natural means of weight loss, that will work without much effort! While during the 'olden times', these berries were more preferred to be taken raw, today they come in different forms, including juices and supplements.

The berry, also called the "Beauty berry" in Brazil, was found to be full of natural energy and also rich in all proteins, minerals, omega oils and vitamins like Vitamin E, which would help to keep a person's body and immune system under check. It was also known for its ability to control prostate enlargement.

It is also said to offer some similarities to the benefits of Viagra. After the qualities of these berries began to be known to the common man, people, especially the beach boys even began to use the crushed and refrigerated pulp of these berries while enjoying special holidays with their partners!

But the biggest problem in using these berries was that they had a very short lifespan of 24 hours, when the richness and the qualities of the berry would remain. The possibilities of eating the berries raw, so as to take advantage of its qualities, thus became limited, owing to the processes involved in getting the berries from the palms, transportation etc. But soon, researchers found a way to overcome these problems and to make these berries available for us. They developed these berries into a more easily consumable and available form for the market – the Acai berry supplement.

Coming in the form of supplements, these berries have the power not only to boost your immunity but also to fight infections and to provide protection to your heart. Now, you may be wondering how can such a supplement help reduce heart disease. The fact is that the ratio of fatty acids in the Acai berry is almost similar to that of olive oil, which is well known for its ability to control heart disease, over normal oils. This is the same reason why the supplements made from these berries can help you keep your heart protected. The supplements are actually an easier means to consume it, for people who do not wish to experience the vibrant berry taste that has little sweetness and is not really very appetizing.

Apart from the pills, there is also the Acai berry powder, which can be used as a supplement to promote weight loss. This powder is readily available in the market today and is quite easy to consume. All you need to do is take a few spoons of this powder, add it to water or milk, mix well and then drink! As simple as that!

If you are a person looking to buy the Acai berry diet supplement for weight loss, you needn't search around a lot. They are usually available in the form of capsules and can be purchased without any prescription, which is indeed the biggest advantage. All you need to do is find a store near your locality that sells these precious little capsules. It is not just the Acai berry alone, which causes your weight loss. Instead, there are other important components too in this supplement, which work together synergistically with the berries to make weight loss possible.

Using these supplements is not just about weight loss. The fact is that not only will you be able to lose weight, but your immune system tends to become stronger, which means that you won't be affected by harmful molecules and radicals that can cause serious diseases.

Studies also indicate that the Acai berry has the ability to fight and kill cancer cells, due to the fact that it is one of the best antioxidant berries available today, even stronger than ginkgo biloba, which had been known for its high medicinal properties for more than a thousand years. So, from this, what is to be understood is that, by taking an Acai berry supplement, you are not just making your immune system stronger, but you are making yourself less prone to deadly cancers!

Today, these supplements are highly popular among the stars as well as average people, as a simple means of weight loss and in keeping the immune system strong so we stay protected from diseases.

There are a lot of supplements available on the market today with the Acai berry as their main ingredient. The Brazilian Acai berry is one such supplement that is very popular. Studies reveal that the Brazilian Acai berry is currently being used by many Hollywood stars and individuals from all over the world who are trying to lose weight in a safe and effective manner.

Good Acai berry supplements often include more than just the extract from the Acai berry, they offer green tea, chromium polynicotinate, gymnema sylvestre, caffeine and garcinia cambogia as their main ingredients, which together help to increase the metabolic rate of the body. This achieves a substantial and progressive weight loss as compared to other supplements, minimizing the conversion of carbohydrates into body fats, bringing about increased energy levels and controlled blood sugar and many more advantages for the human body.

The chief advantage of this supplement is that you will be able to gain all these health benefits without much effort or tedious work! However, for those people who have issues in using caffeine or products with caffeine, this supplement may not be a good suggestion.

Where would you go for some such supplements? Owing to the increase in demand, today there a lot of companies selling the Acai berry supplements. But are all of them the real Acai berry supplements? When you have decided to pay for these supplements, you need to make sure that you get your hands on the right ones, rather than the fake ones, which are available along with the real ones.

The first thing to check for when you are about to buy these supplements is the content provided. You need to make sure that the major ingredient of the supplement you are about to buy is the Acai berry itself. If you do a thorough search, you may find that there are many supplements that come under the title Acai berry supplements, but its major ingredients is something else, which you may not need for your specific condition.

The products from different companies may vary in their ingredients. It is up to you, to choose the one that fits your requirements. The next thing you need to look at is the price. Cheaper ones may be available on the market but make sure that they are genuine before jumping in and buying them. If both these check out, you should do fairly well in buying a good bottle of these berry supplements!

How the Supplement Works and Results in Weight Loss

Now that we have gone through the history and details of the Acai berry and the diet supplements that contain their extracts, let us grab some more details about how it works to reduce weight and boost your immune system.

People call the Acai berry a super-food. This is because it consists of a whole lot of nutrients, minerals, and vitamins which help in managing the whole of your body well enough to keep it healthy and young. The Acai berry is known to consist of natural ingredients that boost your metabolic rate. A boost in the metabolic rate of your body can cause the use of more calories to get your daily tasks done. This, in turn, results in your body burning excess fat faster.

The fiber content in these supplements also tends to reduce your craving of eating, by giving you a feeling of a full stomach. The reduced intake of food also helps in reducing the weight of the body by a good amount.

Studies reveal that the antioxidants in Acai berries cleanses your body, kidneys and liver from any toxic materials that you may have consumed, thereby making your body stronger and resistant to diseases. Some of these antioxidants include anthocyanins and homoorientin.

Now how do these toxic substances enter your body? The fact is that your normal metabolic activities can cause the formation of some toxic substances within the body. Along with this, exposure to cigarette smoke, polluted air etc. can also result in the inhalation of toxic substances as well. These substances cause the formation of free radicals, which in turn leads to degeneration of our cells, causing damages and diseases. The strong antioxidants in the Acai berry allow more flow of oxygen into the body and destroy these free radicals, thereby making cell growth possible. This in turn makes you stronger and tougher against all diseases.

Apart from this, the berry is known to consist of rare nutrients and monounsaturated fats. They are also one of the few fruits that contain these unique types of fats. It is a well-known fact that monounsaturated fats are very beneficial when it comes to dieting and losing weight quickly. Acai berries consist of several nutrients such as iron, calcium, and even different vitamins that are vital for the body, including Vitamin A, Vitamin C etc., which promotes betterment of the skin, enhanced vision and so many more qualities that help to keep you younger and more active, even at old age!

Research Conducted

After the advantages of using the Acai berry started to gain popularity, several researches and studies were conducted on it, to prove the antioxidant abilities of the berry in fighting cancer cells, increasing the energy level of the body etc. And miraculously, these studies and researches conducted helped to show the fact that Acai berries possess the ability to destroy dangerous cancer cells, provide more energy to the body and boost one's immune system.

In the year 2006, Florida University conducted a research on the abilities of the Acai berry to kill cancer causing cells. The university was one among the first to research the advantages of the Acai berry. The experienced personnel of the University including Stephen Talcott, Susan Percival and David Del conducted the researches on the Acai berry and its cancer killing abilities. The research was conducted on cultured cancer cells and it was found that after the use of the berries on these cancer cells, the cells began to die. Talcott described this study as an important part in learning how these Acai supplements, juice and the berries themselves can be of use to the mankind.

But these results weren't completely backed by the researchers. This was because the research was done on cultured cancer cells and not real ones. And for this reason, the researchers did not wish to spread a false hope about a natural treatment for this disastrous disease! Moreover, the study pointed to the fact that the effect of such antioxidants on the growth of cancer cells were influenced by many other factors, like the metabolism rate, nutrient absorption etc. Hence, coming to a complete conclusion that the Acai berries can prevent the attack of cancer fully became probable.

The University of Florida also conducted another research towards the end of 2006, regarding the antioxidant effect of the

Acai berries on healthy individuals. The intention of this study was to understand the rate at which the blood absorbs the compounds, and their effects on the cholesterol levels, blood pressure etc. of a person.

In 2008, a study was conducted by the University of Texas to examine the health benefits of acai berry. Twelve healthy volunteers were chosen and were asked to consume just one serving of the Acai berry in pulp or juice form. Urine and blood samples were then taken from all the volunteers after a break of 12 hours and 24 hours.

It was found that all the volunteers experienced an increase in their antioxidant activity and an improvement in their immunity system. This research led to the need for further research studies to determine what the real health benefits of the berry are and the disease fighting abilities it may possess. The researchers suggested that these should be determined so as to estimate the amount of Acai berry pulp, juice or its supplements that should be consumed by a person, to get the best results. But they did not fully conclude that this berry is an 'all disease fighter' - yet. The researchers concluded with a doubt, if this berry may be just a part of a good balanced diet and not the balanced diet itself. Studies are still being conducted on the benefits of the Acai berries and the other qualities it may possess, which in turn can be a breakthrough in the treatment of several diseases and ailments.

Ingredients

There are various ingredients in this weight loss supplement you should be aware of such as:

•Acai berry (4:1 concentrate): Acai berry is the most important ingredient in this weight loss supplement. Acai berries consist of anthocyanins which is an antioxidant that decreases cholesterol levels. Acai berries consist of plant sterols that improve cardiovascular health and enhance blood circulation. Research conducted in the Rio de Janeiro University proved that consuming Acai berries on a regular basis can help in weight loss and improve your health as well.

•Cascara Sagrada (10% extract): Cascara Sagrada is one of the most important ingredients in the Brazilian acai berry weight loss supplement and is also given the name Persian bark. It has been used for hundreds of centuries now as a natural purgative. It is mainly used as a tonic for inflamed gallstones and enhances bile secretion. It can also be used to treat enlarged livers and problems in the digestion system.

•Senna Leaves (6% extract): Senna leaves are unique shrubs that grow in Egypt and are collected two times per year. They are then dried out to create various medicinal tea and supplements. These leaves are very beneficial on your health especially when it comes to smoothing muscles in the colon and stabilizing bowel movements. It is mainly used in medicines for colon problems and constipation.

•Black Walnut (herb powder): Black walnuts are very beneficial for the arteries and veins because they decrease inflammation and eliminate substances that end up in blocking arteries. They are also used to treat problems in the circulatory system, asthma, and decrease your risk of suffering from cancer. Black walnuts have laxative properties as well and can improve problems in the digestion system and colon.

•Bentonite Clay: What a lot of people aren't aware of is that Bentonite clay is originally volcanic ash that has aged. It has been used for years now to treat different medical conditions. It has other health benefits as well as cleansing the colon, balancing bacteria, improving the assimilation of nutrients in your body and improving the immune system. Additionally, bentonite clay is used for treating food poisoning and allergies.

Recommended dosage

When you take Brazilian acai berry on a daily basis, you can expect to lose around five pounds per week. However, you should always remember that this will differ from one person to another. The effects of this supplement will also increase if you consume a healthy diet and exercise. Keep in mind that good acai supplements consists of special types of herbs and ingredients that will fasten the weight loss process.

The price of the supplement will differ from one company to another. The cheapest supplement will cost you around $15 per bottle and you will find around sixty tablets in it. It is recommended to take two capsules per day but this will differ from one person to another.

Your best choice would be to consult a doctor, before adding such supplements to your daily diet. An over dosage of these supplements can cause diarrhea. If this happens, just cut back. You may also have allergic reactions, depending on how your body reacts to berries and the other ingredients in the supplement. If any reaction occurs, it would be best if you stop consuming the supplements further and check with a doctor immediately.

Benefits of the Brazilian Acai Berry Supplement

•A part from what was stated above, Acai has very few or no side effects whatsoever. The fact remains that it is a simple berry available naturally from the forests. Studies reveal that these berries were in use hundreds of years ago as a means of increasing one's energy level and even as a cure from many diseases. The fact that these berries can be taken fresh or in the pulped form or even as juices, without adding any chemical to them supports the statement that there are very few or no side effects at all for these berries or supplements made from them.

Although, one of the possible side effects may arise from the caffeine, which is one of the ingredients in a few of the Acai berry diet supplements available in the market. For those people who cannot intake caffeine, these products are better to be avoided. There are also chances of slight diarrhea, if the pills or supplements are taken in excess quantity. Studies also reveal that those people who have pollen allergies may have problems and allergic reactions to such berries or the supplements made from it.

•Enables you to lose weight easily – For those people who are tired of spending countless hours in your life, trying to burn out the excess fat in your body, the Acai berry supplements would be worth trying. Instead of spending long hours doing exercises, you just need to make the Acai berries or its juice or even the Acai berry supplements, a mandatory part of your daily diet. The ability of the Acai berry supplements to limit the conversion of the carbohydrates you consume into body fat is the main aid in keeping your body weight under control.

This supplement tends to stabilize your body sugar and bring down the bad cholesterol in your body, while promoting the increase in good cholesterol level. Moreover, they increase your metabolism rate, which causes the use of more calories to burn in your body daily. This, in turn, helps you lose weight and keep your body weight under check, that too, without much effort! The role of the fiber contained in the Acai berry supplements should also not be overlooked. The contents when eaten, tend to fill your stomach to your satisfaction, which in turn reduces the amount of food consumed for a day. That is, it acts as a hunger suppressant. And that, of course, aids in quick weight loss!

•The supplement is very affordable compared to other products – When you are out to purchase the Acai berry supplements, you will find that they are much less expensive than competitor diet supplements available in the market today. If you are planning on buying them online, you may find even cheaper deals compared to buying them directly from shops. But then, you need to be careful about the quality of the product you buy.

Like every other product, these diet supplements and powders can also have fake and cheap look-alikes in the market! If you do a thorough search, you can see that there are companies that sell these products for prices around $24 for a 4 oz. bag. This can last you for around a dozen or more juices made from these berries. And after the discounts, special offers etc. which they offer, you can get your precious supplements for prices as low as $14! This is of course very cheap, if you compare it to other costly products and procedures that promote weight loss, but yet don't work a bit!

•Slows down aging – The Acai berries have not only been known for their weight loss properties, but they have also been well-known from long ago for their ability to bring about youthfulness to one's skin. The women and men of years ago used to eat these berries to keep themselves fresh and young. The fact is that these berries aided in increasing one's sexual desire, something that keeps a human being full of life, no matter what age he or she is!

Moreover, the anti-oxidant properties of the berries made them the best choice in the search for a natural anti-aging product. One of the main anti-oxidants in the Acai Berry, called anthocyanins, is expected to be the cause of the anti-aging properties of the Acai berry. Today, these berries are being used not only in diet supplements but also in beauty products, including anti-aging creams and other cosmetic items, owing to the anti-aging properties they possess.

How exactly do they slow down aging? These berries are rich in flavonoids, which help in fighting inflammations. They also have fatty acids, amino acids etc., which act with these flavonoids to aid in the regenerative growth of one's skin cells. Moreover, these berries contain a significant amount of nutrients that help to keep one's skin and body healthy and glowing. It is not just about slowing down aging. These berries in the beauty products help to absorb moisture into your skin and aid in the removal of blemishes, skin infections etc., which in turn helps to give a better tone to your skin. It is even said to protect you from the harmful UV rays of the sun as well as other stressors that might harm your skin and cause quick aging.

•Enhanced cardiovascular health – The Acai berry supplements are known to have the ability to protect your heart from diseases and keep it healthy. How is this achieved? The main reason for this property of these supplements is that they contain a lot of herbal ingredients that can directly and indirectly aid in protecting your heart. The health of your heart has a lot to do with the level of fats and cholesterol in your body. With its beneficial properties that aid in the reduction of bad cholesterol and burning of calories, Acai berry supplements reduce the chances of a person to be prone to heart diseases and other cardiovascular problems. The berries and its supplements also have the ability to reduce the blood pressure of your body. Studies reveal that taking the Acai berry supplements can bring down your chances of suffering from a stroke by a huge percentage.

•Enhances the digestion process – The ability of the Acai berry supplements to speed up the metabolism of the human body is the secret behind this. The fatty acids, omega acids etc. present in the Acai berries aid in better metabolic rates and along with this, causes the speeding up of the digestion of food that is being consumed.

•Improves blood circulation and cholesterol levels – Due to the ability of the Acai berries to vary the cholesterol level in the body. Diet supplements containing the Acai berry also have this same healthy benefit. The reduction in the amount of bad cholesterol and the increase in the amount of good cholesterol in the body help in keeping the cholesterol levels at check and preventing excess fats in getting deposited in the body. The nutrients, minerals etc. present in the berry are the major contributors of increased blood circulation throughout our body, which in turn, leads to an increase in our total energy level, at no matter what age! Moreover, these supplements tend to detoxify and clean up our system, thereby making our body better and healthier in all manner of ways.

•Decreases joint pain – This is very beneficial for individuals who suffer from arthritis and other similar problems. How is this achieved? As mentioned above, these supplements aid in better circulation of the blood throughout the body, which in turn helps in relaxing your muscles and reducing joint pains. For those who have constant joint pains, muscle pains etc., the Acai berry supplements can turn out to be a good medicine that gives relief from their constant pains. Taking this supplement will also improve the condition of your muscles and enhance the process of muscle regeneration, which is great for body builders and those who exercise.

•Improves sex drive – Sex drive is something that keeps a man and woman young and fresh, no matter what age they are. It is a known fact that the sex drive decreases in most people, with the increase in age and this is one of the major reasons that cause you to look aged physically. Even from ancient times, the Acai berry was known to have a good effect on the sexual desire of a human being. Studies revealed that taking the pulp of these berries could help in enhancing your sex drive regardless of your age. Today the Acai berry supplements are being used not only as a means of weight loss but also secretly to increase sex drive and bring about a better interest in one's partner. This has particularly been very beneficial for those individuals who have an unstable sexual relationship with their partner and those people who have been experiencing trouble in their married life.

•The variety of products available and ease of availability – Ranging from fresh pulp to diet powders and pills, the Acai berry is widely available in the market today. You just need to search around the nearest shops or even online, to purchase them for affordable rates. These berries have been introduced into bars and other snack products and you can see them on sale even in gymnasiums and other common stores.

The Acai berry juice is also readily available in many stores, if you wish to consume a fresher and more direct version of the berry. On other hand, if it is an easy method you are looking for, you can opt for the diet powders and supplements containing the Acai berries. The Brazilian Acai berry is just one among the many best Acai berry products available in the market today. If you haven't tried it, then you are definitely missing a lot. There are thousands of people who are using it right now with the best results of achieving good weight loss and getting back into normal shape with these supplements!

•Boost to your immune system – Resistance to diseases is something we all possess right from the time we are born. But the level of immunity in each individual may vary according his body, eating habits etc. The Acai berry diet supplements are said to be the best friends of those people who have a weak immune system. Why is the Acai berry good for your immune system?

Studies reveal that the Acai berries grew in tough conditions and were exposed to a lot of sunlight, due to the height of the Acai palms. So as to overcome the harmful effects of sunrays, Nature itself is said to have given these berries a huge supply of antioxidants which would provide more oxygen and would help the berry exist in these tough conditions. The anti-oxidant powers of the berries are suspected to be the real causes to the boost in the immune system of the person eating them. It has been found that these anti-oxidants in the Acai berries have the strong ability to destroy or kill the free radicals and aid in the healing of any damaged cell in the human body. Hence, the Acai berry diet supplements are also said to possess these powers of strengthening your immune system and making you less prone to diseases, unlike many other diet supplements which promote weight loss.

•Ability to fight cancer cells – As mentioned before, the strong anti-oxidant properties of the Acai berry supplements are said to aid in destroying cancer cells to an extent. The berries are known to have 5 times better anti-oxidant properties compared to the best anti-oxidants known to man today and this is expected to become a breakthrough in the treatment of cancer, if proven true. Although research is being conducted on this and a clear statement is not yet possible that these supplements can prevent cancer from attacking a human body completely, it may soon come. Better safe than sorry and take them now.

Having discussed about the qualities of the Acai berry and the supplements made from it, now it is time for you to decide if you wish to make use of this simple super-food to make yourself younger and more energetic! Go ahead, try it out at least once and feel the difference in just days. Say goodbye to tiring workouts and welcome to Acai berries!

Important Tips for Increasing the Supplements' Effect

Just like any other weight loss supplement, you shouldn't except to lose any weight or some kind of miracle if you continue in eating junk food or neglect exercising. Even though these outstanding diet supplements are designed in a way to help you in losing weight, eating the wrong types of food will increase the amount of toxins in your body. When this happens, your body will want to automatically protect itself by increasing the amount of fats surrounding your tissue and organs.

When you use raspberry ketones, it is recommended that you follow a special fitness program so you can reach the desired effects at a faster rate. Recommended exercises include walking or jogging every morning. If you have a busy schedule, you can look for exercises that can be performed from the convenience of your own home.

Many people have little exercise equipment and no gym membership. There are many things we can do in our own home to lose weight and get in shape that cost nothing. If you have a computer with an Internet connection, you can lookup many sites that offer great home workouts. This is one that many women (and men), who are new to exercising are following, www.robinskey.com, which offers lots of exercise videos to follow. It's totally free and I only recommend it because it works, and because Robin, the person behind it, is totally genuine. To go directly to her videos, visit https://www.youtube.com/user/robinkeikogregory

Drinking water every day can also help you in losing weight at a faster rate and this will also ensure that your skin will stay hydrated and shiny all the time. You should try to drink at least eight cups of water each day to reach the desired effects. These tips are very important to follow because many people think that all they have to do is follow the diet and it will work like magic. There is no way that the diet will work successfully if you eat food that if rich in fats all the time or don't exercise enough.

Here are some guidelines you can follow to ensure that you will reach the desired effect and lose weight quickly:

•When you wake up in the morning, the first thing you should do is drink one cup of water or fresh juice. It is recommended to drink juice that consists of vitamin C, such as lemon or orange juice. This will ensure that your body will stay cleansed throughout the day.

•The next thing you should do is eat a breakfast that is healthy to ensure that you will have energy all day. This will ensure that you will have energy especially if you eat a breakfast that consists of fibers, whole grains or low fat protein.

•You should then take one pill of your weight loss supplement right after breakfast.

•If you have time, you should try exercising for at least thirty minutes per day. You should try as much as possible to find an exercise that you enjoy so you don't get bored or feel lazy. Some of the exercises you can perform include walking and jogging. There are many people who purchased treadmills or other types of equipment so they can be able to exercise freely at home, especially if they have very busy schedules or lifestyles.

•If you feel hungry throughout the day, then you should eat small snacks, such as a mix of vegetables or yoghurt.

•At night, try to have a healthy dinner such as grilled chicken or a salad. You should never eat three hours before you go to sleep.

•After dinner, you should take the second dosage of your weight loss supplement unless it says to take 30 minutes before meals.

This may differ from one weight loss supplement to another. For example, you should take the green coffee bean extract three times per day and not two. If this is the case, you should take one in the morning, afternoon, and at night.

If you know someone that is trying to lose weight as well, then you should try going through this process together. One of the most important aspects of losing weight is patience and motivation. When you have someone with you that is trying to lose weight and reach the same goal, you will motivate each other all the time and this is very beneficial so that you don't feel stressed out, hopeless, or tired. For example, you can both remind each other if you miss a dosage of one of the weight loss supplements or you can go walking or jogging every morning together. Each of you can keep the other accountable.

You should try as much as possible to set a goal for yourself. Even though losing weight depends on whether you follow the weight loss supplement directions properly and whether you follow up with exercising and a proper diet, setting a goal yourself will ensure that you won't be demotivated or get lazy. For example, set a goal of losing five pounds per week or per month, and check by the end that period whether you reached that or not.

It is also essential that you remember that the dosage might differ from one person to another. This is very important because many people complain that they didn't lose weight like other people when they took one of the weight loss supplements. You should always remember that we all have different body shapes and health conditions and there is no way a weight loss supplement will work the same way for everyone, no matter how effective it is. If you are unsure of the dosage you should take, try to consult a doctor before you start following the diet. The most important thing is for you to follow the dosage exactly as it is prescribed for you on a daily basis.

Other Companies that Provide the Same Supplement

Due to most of these weight loss supplements consisting of ingredients that are very rare, you will find that many companies sell them for a very expensive price. High quality weight loss supplements will cost you $60 and you might find them for as high as $315. It is recommended that you purchase the supplement from sellers who are acclaimed and reputable. Even though the FDA approved the supplement, this doesn't mean that there are various scammers who will sell you an empty version of the supplement. There are some factors you need to examine before you make a purchase such as:

•The Cost – Even though some of these supplements are a bit more expensive than other products, you need to make sure that you are paying for the correct and genuine product. For example, every single person would like to purchase the cheapest product possible, but this doesn't mean that you will get the best raspberry ketone supplement. There are various scams going on right now and the fact that many people are just looking for a product that is cheap is making things worse. You should make sure that you are receiving what you are paying for regarding the dosage and the size of the bottle.

•The Seller – The source you make a purchase from has to be credible and reputable. You should take your time in researching the source you are making a purchase from to avoid getting disappointed. It is very important that you look out for offers that provide you with a free trial. Even though a few of them might be credible, you will find out that most of them are actually scams. Most of these trials are extremely hard to unsubscribe to or cancel and will consist of low doses, or unoriginal raspberry ketones. This is very important because many people assume that just because all the companies advertise the same product, they will all work the same exact way.

•The Ingredients – The number one reason behind the success of these weight loss supplements is the ingredients they have in them. The diet consists of natural, organic, and healthy ingredients that enable individuals to lose weight and consists of antioxidants that are beneficial for your health and body as well. For example, when it comes to the raspberry ketones diet, there are some ingredients in this diet that need to be included such as raspberry ketone enzymes, acai berry, and green tea. If your supplement doesn't consist of these ingredients, then you should consider looking for another supplier that does. The combination of ingredients in this diet is very important and they are the main reason behind weight loss. There is no point purchasing a diet that doesn't consist of the ingredients that you need.

Conclusion

You have probably understood by now how beneficial these supplements are to weight loss and your overall health. As mentioned previously, you should never forget to use the diet in its proper recommended dosages and combine it with exercising and healthy food choices. Losing weight has never been easier and your energy and metabolism will increase as well, something that doesn't happen with other supplements. This is definitely great because you will be able to gain various health benefits other than losing weight. It is essential that you consume the diet exactly as it is recommended for you. Even though we all want to lose weight at a fast rate, taking the wrong dosage may not be beneficial to your health and you won't lose weight any faster. If you have been overweight for a long time, then this is definitely the best solution in the market right now for you. There isn't any other supplement in the market that will enable you to lose weight in a safe and effective manner like the ones mentioned in this book.